JENNY BEEK[EN]

DON'T
HOLD
YOUR
BREATH

ILLUSTRATED BY
JANITA STENHOUSE

POLAIR PUBLISHING · LONDON

First Published by Polair Publishing, November 2004

British Library Cataloguing-in-Publication Data
A catalogue record for this book is available from the British Library

ISBN 0-95452389-9-4

Acknowledgments
I am grateful to Pauline Sawyer and Sue Peggs, for their inspiration.
I should also like to thank Janita Stenhouse, for considerable co-operation in the
preparation of the illustrations, Louise Pagliaro, who typed the manuscript, and Katherine Haw, who
proofread the book. Thanks are also due to Wildwood House, Ltd., for permission to use the text of
the Mandukya Upanishad on pp. 29–30, and to the publishers of the other short extracts whose details
are given, along with the quotations, in the text.

Printed in Great Britain by
Cambridge University Press

CONTENTS

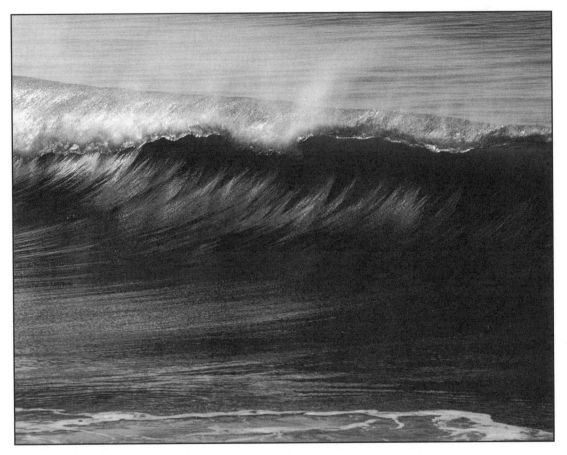

INTRODUCTION

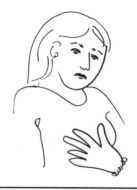

> *There is a difference between a calm, conscious breath that gives lightness to the body and clarity to the mind and a short, mechanical one that cripples the body and dulls the mind.*
>
> Sandra Sabatini

'DON'T hold your breath' is an expression usually associated with waiting in excitement and anticipation for something which is not really expected to happen. Yet most of us hold our breath a lot of the time. Is that in anticipation of something that really *is* going to happen, or is it something else?

What is it that makes us hold our breath? We are going to investigate that in this book. Generally, it is something that makes us either fearful or excited, but it may be something that totally intrigues us. It may also have become a habit.

When they are distracted by fears, fascination or excitement, people forget to breathe. Some people breathe in and hold their breath in, while other people breathe out and then keep the breath out. To do either is connected with how our minds and our emotions work and reflects in our energy; gradually, it can create a lot of problems in our health. By giving close attention to how we breath and when we breath, by being conscious of the pattern of

5

our breath, we can understand our whole system much better. By being aware of our breath and allowing it to function naturally, we can find a lot more energy, as well as harmony and balance. We can also significantly improve our health.

Just about everybody has an irregular pattern in their breathing. This is because of the unnatural way our lives are led today and because of the strains we put ourselves under in modern life. All of those strains are exactly reflected in the breath. Living in awareness of our breathing, we would probably do many of the same things that we already do but in a much more harmonious way. Looking at the patterns of our breathing can enable us to break habits: not just those which are in our breathing, but also ones in our lives. They are precisely the habits that do not enable us to live a harmonious, satisfied, well-balanced life. With some practice, some awareness of our breath, we can change absolutely how we are. By a gradual undoing of patterning, we change how we feel, how we relate to people and how our life is.

Attention and investigation are needed over time, as what we have to deal with are usually long-held habits, often copied from our parents. They may have created much disharmony in our lives. As we become aware of them, the better patterns slowly enable us to live a full, contented, enlivened life.

This book contains many methods of bringing awareness to your breath, to how the breath moves through the body and what you can do with it. Most of these are simple, and are drawn from yoga, but you don't need already to be a yoga student to use this book.

The yoga practice of awareness of the breath is called *pranayama*. The direct translation of *prana* is primary energy, often called the vital life-force. Among students of yoga, there is much debate as to whether this is the air itself or something contained in the air. Yet yoga also has a vocabulary which western science lacks for a more subtle level at which such an energy can work. This is the level of the breath body, what yoga calls the *prana maya kosa* (*maya* means illusion, or another level from what we call our level of reality, and *kosa* means veil or sheath). Through the breath body, the air connects with every cell in our body. Truly conscious breathing also brings into focus the cellular breathing we do, notably through the skin, until every cell pulsates with life.

Ayama, the other half of the word *pranayama*, means expansion—expansion of the life-force. *Ayama* has also been translated as control, which might seem to imply forcing your breathing in some way. Yet by our just bringing attention to our breath it deepens naturally. It lengthens and so expands the amount of the life-force in us.

It is very important not to impose forceful techniques of inhalation and exhalation onto an irregular pattern of breathing. *Pranayama* would then be dangerous. I am not wanting the practices in this book to be forceful, so please don't take them to the point of strain. They are given to enhance your normal breathing pattern, so that your everyday life is more joyful, more peaceful, more full of love and lived with more sense of ease and acceptance of its ups and downs. Your breath exactly reflects how you react to it.

The *Hatha Yoga Pradipika*, the classic yoga text, gives instruction in the techniques of breathing very forcefully—and then states that they all such techniques come naturally with practice. I have found this to be true, but real naturalness comes over literally years of practice, so a great deal of perseverance is needed.

STARTING TO WORK ON YOUR BREATH

To start, can you actually feel yourself breathing in? Can you feel what is needed in the body for the breath to find its way in? Does your ribcage move? Does your breastbone move at all?

Then, what do you notice moving in your body as you breathe out? Moreover, do you breathe in and then stop, breathe out and then stop, or is it continuous apart from a tiny moment at the end of each half of the breath where it stands still? Do you rush the breath out? Do you draw it in forcefully, or can it come in at its own pace?

All the things mentioned put a strain on your body, your breath and your feeling self. One of the most helpful ways of getting some rhythm back into your breathing is to sit by the sea and breathe so as to copy the rhythm of the sea. Feel the movement of the air coming into your lungs as the water comes up to the crest of the wave, opening your lungs further all the way. Then feel the tumbling over of the wave as you go into the exhalation. There is a natural pause at the beginning and end of both halves of the movement, both with your breath and with the wave.

You can, of course, use the pictures in this book and listen to the wave in your imagination, rather than watching an actual sea; or listen to gentle surge on the shore.

Notice whether you breathe through your mouth or through your nose. If it is more through your mouth, what does it feel like to breathe a little more through the nostrils? This may not be easy and need some practice, so don't force the pace, but as you use this book try gradually to develop the habit of breathing through your nose.

Now work through the book at your own pace. You will discover which sections are most helpful.

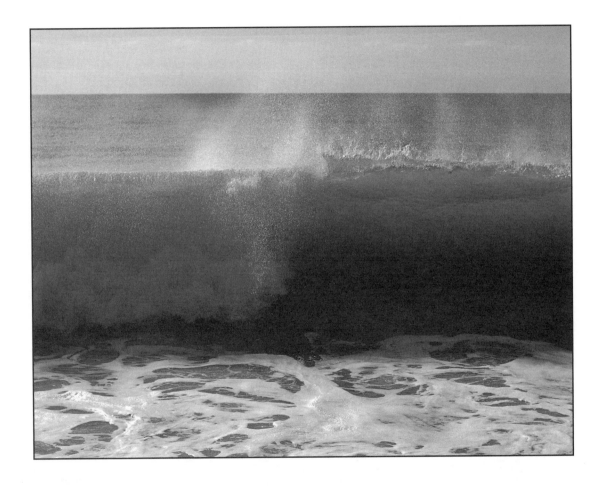

CHAPTER ONE
Do *You* Hold your Breath?

DO YOU hold your breath half of the time? Did you realize some people hold their breath in, while others hold it out?

Typically, those of us who tend constantly to be rushing around, trying to do a great deal in their

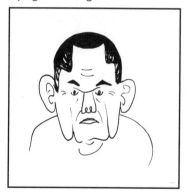

lives, are the ones who breathe in and then hold their breath there. They forget to breathe out, or even feel they haven't got time to do so. They thus push themselves through life on an inbreath. Theirs tend to be lives lived in a constant pattern of stress.

Does this sound all too familiar to you? Do you notice, if you sit or lie down, that it's only then that you take a full breath? Or in the general pattern of life, when you are faced with a situation where you feel a quick response is needed from you, where you are under scrutiny, or when you are expected to do something decisively, efficiently or well, do you notice that you are holding your breath in the moment you try to do that? Does it feel that were you to breathe out for a moment nothing would get done—that you would literally deflate? Nothing would happen, perhaps, and you would be going nowhere? Is this the belief of eve-

ryone that holds their breath in?

On the other hand, there are the people who hold their breath out and then don't feel the ability to breathe in. Maybe they have a belief that life is not fulfilling for them, not giving them what they need or

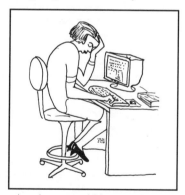

what they want. We may ask, what is the point of taking a full breath if life doesn't sustain us, doesn't nurture us? You may notice this in

DISEASES ASSOCIATED WITH HOLDING THE BREATH IN	DISEASES ASSOCIATED WITH HOLDING THE BREATH OUT
High blood-pressure, heart disease, tension, migraine, headaches, angina; all stress-related diseases.	Low blood-pressure, multiple sclerosis, depression, M.E. (fatigue syndrome), lack of energy for life.

yourself if you feel dull, depressed, or lacking energy. In these circumstances, do you tend to breathe out and then come upon a moment of feeling that you can't take breath in, you can't take life in?

Don't worry if one or other of these patterns seems to apply to you. Don't get alarmed, either, if you think you may suffer from one of the diseases mentioned in the boxes. This book is here to help!

We are going to do something about breathing patterns in the next exercises. They are what we shall call 'practices', because they are like ongoing exercises, things you can do all the time.

Breath is life, the basic and most fundamental expression of our life. In Judaism ruah, the breath, means the spirit of God that infuses the creation; in Christianity also there is a profound link between the Holy Spirit, without which nothing could have life, and the breath. In the teaching of Buddha, the breath, or prana in Sanskrit, is said to be 'the vehicle of the mind', because it is the prana that makes our mind move. So when you calm the mind by working skilfully with the breath, you are simultaneously and automatically taming and training the mind. Haven't we all experienced how relaxing it can be when life is stressful, to be alone for a few minutes and just breathe, in and out, deeply and quietly? Even such a simple exercise can help us a great deal.
Sogyal Rinpoche, MEDITATION *(Rider, London, 1994)*

POSTURES TO ENCOURAGE BREATHING

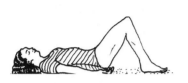
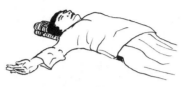
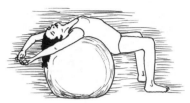

PREPARATION

IT IS helpful to start most of the breathing practices in this book lying down (the exceptions are individually noted). You then feel the breath more into the back part of the body. The back of the body can also 'spread' more at the start if you bend the knees and spread the feet down, as in the left-hand drawing above. 'Spreading' is a term I have defined elsewhere as being like softening, relaxing, with the feeling that the part in question can take up more space.

This position is sometimes called the effortless pose. The arms should spread out and down. In this relaxed position, the eyes can gently look down. Other things

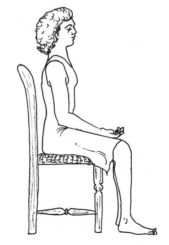

that can be helpful are spreading the ribs at the side, and lifting the upper back on blocks or a folded blanket, or using an exercise ball.

Feel the tailbone lengthen away towards your feet and down towards the ground. This minute movement of the tailbone lengthens the whole spine, right from the crown, while easing it out like a string of pearls. (The vertebrae are actually likened to a string of pearls in ancient yoga texts.)

If you prefer to sit, rather than lie down, the spine needs to be upright so that the ribcage is open. All the upper body should be relaxed, not straightened by tensing.

The posture has a significant and immediate effect on the breathing.

If you are already a yoga student, Shri B. K. S. Iyengar recommends that you practise the *asanas* to prepare your body for *pranayama*, The *asanas* lengthen the spine out, and they lift the breastbone up and spread the back body to help you breathe. Preparation in this way will itself change your breathing before you even begin *pranayama*. It is very difficult to breathe differently from normal if the spine is collapsed down, or if the upper back or the shoulders are hunched in, or if the breastbone caved in.

Suitable postures in which breathing practice can be done and felt include sitting cross-legged. In the left-hand illustration, where sitting back to back with another person is a way of helping the spine lengthen and feel supported, you may notice that while the left-hand person sits cross-legged, the right-hand one is shown in the yoga pose *virasana*, hero: kneeling but with the feet outside the buttocks, which are supported by a blanket.

The other pictures show *baddha konasana*, cobbler pose, where the soles of the feet are together. If it's a strain to stretch the spine up in this posture, then sit against a wall with a rolled blanket across the top of the sacrum and in the lumbar region (as in the right-hand picture), to allow the natural curve of the lumbar spine, resting the backs of the hands on the knees and opening the shoulders out.

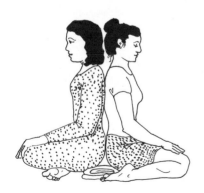
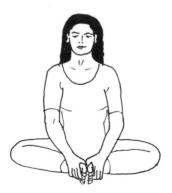
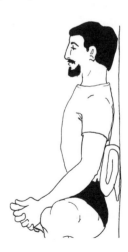

PRACTICE 1 : VILOMA (LADDER BREATH) ON THE EXHALATION

A BREATH which you take in stages, further and further into you, or one which you expel bit by bit, is known as a ladder breath. If you are aware of your breathing in, and feel relatively happy about how you do it, but don't always find it so easy to breathe out or feel you don't do so completely, then to do a few of these on the exhalation is a good practice for you.

Sit comfortably or lie down with your spine lengthened out and your breastbone spread (as described in the section on preparation, p, 11). Feel the breath come and go, without doing anything special, for a few breaths—until the pattern of your breath naturally lengthens and deepens. This will happen merely from your observation of it. Now, aware of the air as you do it, gently breathe in. Breathe out just a little, then pause.

Exhale a bit more, and then pause; and then exhale again and repeat

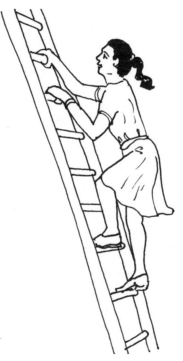

until you feel you have breathed right out. It is rather as though the breath is going out in little wavelets, with a rest or pause in between them. You may find at the beginning you make just a couple of pauses, and then let the breath come in again.

Feel how much more easily and deeply the air comes in after you have done this a few times. Do you open more to the breath as it comes in? Then exhale a little, pause; exhale, pause—throughout the exhalation, as though you are coming down the body step by step, stepping down a ladder. Let the breath come in again when it is ready.

If a sound comes naturally with the exhalation, like a sigh, let this come—so that you exhale with a bit of a sigh, pause, sigh, pause, sigh—until again you have breathed right out. It is a good idea to take a couple of easy breaths in and easy breaths out in between the ladder breaths to relax. If you feel they are demanding, if the exercise is even remotely straining, then don't have so many pauses on the outbreath. You need to feel that you can really breathe in easily after doing this. As you practice, gently and gradually, the exhalation will come to you more naturally.

Increasing experience in what you are doing can lead you on to the stage where you naturally make more of a sound as you do it. Then, rather than exhaling and pausing, you would make a continual sound on the exhalation—like a singer does—recognizing that when you breathe out strongly a sound is produced. Ideally, this sound needs to be a natural one that comes from deep in your belly. If it comes from the throat it will feel strained. Normally, as you make the sound with the air that comes out of your mouth, there will also be an exhalation through the nose that the same time.

Feel as you inhale that you can spread the breath deep into the pelvis. Fill the belly, then fill the ribs, then fill the top part of the chest. Then just let that natural sound, the voice of your own self-expression, come with the exhalation. It will reflect both the underlying you and how you are feeling at the moment. Let it come, however it is: not judging, not seeing what note or what vowel it is, just feeling what sort of sound is there.

Let that sound come, for as much and as many times as feels natural to you. You may want to go where no-one can hear you: may want to sit in the middle of a field to do this or choose to do it when the house is quiet and there is nobody about. You will certainly feel less inhibited when you have some space entirely to yourself. Equally, it is very good to do it in a group. Make sure, though, that you feel always how the inhalation is after this sound, how it really wants to come in and open you and fill you. You may notice that it is easier to exhale afterwards, easier to let the breath go, and may really *feel* that letting go of the exhalation.

When it's difficult to exhale—something we all find at times—what would make you have a really good sigh? What would make you feel *ahhhhh!*—like you could let go totally and breathe out?

With the exhalation, there always needs to be a sense of being able to relax, let go. If you tend to be always on the go, doing a lot and most of the time doing it on a held inhalation, then it is particularly helpful to make a sound through the mouth as you exhale.

Normally, of course, our nose is used for breathing in and breathing out, and our mouth is for eating. Sometimes, however, if it is not easy to breathe out through the nose, it is useful for a while to use the mouth. It is then just as if you are making a sound, singing, talking even—times, obviously, when the mouth is used: you actually *have* to exhale to do that.

Sometimes, problems in breathing out arise from difficulties we may have in saying what we want to say. So we react by holding ourselves in. We hold the breath in, because the sound of ourselves is not being expressed. If you can't really express what you have to say verbally, a sigh or a sound will help in the expression of whatever you are feeling unable to express, even if you can only make this sigh to yourself. In Chapter Four, we ex-

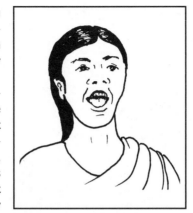

plore using sounds as actual chants.

Making a sound in this way is very therapeutic and releasing. It is helpful if you feel angry or joyful, if you feel frustrated, if you feel sad, if you are bearing grief. That is one reason why in some traditions there are paid mourners at funerals. It helps to lament audibly, to make a sound of showing grief. Singing probably began as a way of expressing emotions like grief—though also joy and love. If you are depressed, again it helps to express the feeling of being depressed in a sound.

Later in this book we look at several conditions that affect our breathing. In each of these, a sound will help the breath, and will help the integration or the relief of the condition if it feels uncomfortable.

PRACTICE 2 : VILOMA (LADDER BREATH) ON THE INHALATION

IF YOU find that you don't breathe *in* easily, then it may be that a ladder breath on the inhalation is what will help.

After breathing out, inhale a little and relax or 'spread' into the belly, the hips, the base area. Pause, but don't hold on at all, don't tense; and then inhale more. Now in your awareness you can come up a little higher: to the top of the pelvis, the sacrum area. Again pause for a second or two, and then inhale more, this time up to the level of the navel. Pause there and inhale yet again, spreading up to the heart and solar plexus area. Feel the breath lifting the heart area. A yoga teacher might refer to the heart chakra or centre, which is the area around the heart.

Inhaling again, bring your awareness up through the top part of the chest so that your throat spreads and relaxes too. Exhale just when

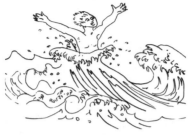

you are ready to, gently and smoothly. You may now need a bit of easy inhalation and exhalation. Just be aware of both: notice how you are breathing, and when you feel ready, again inhale, pause, inhale, pause: travelling up the body as you inhale. Each time you pause, just 'be there' for a moment, and then inhale again, as though the breath is in little waves.

There needs to be no strain, so at the start there may only be a couple of pauses you want to make on the inhalation. But go on breathing easily afterwards, feeling

whether the ladder breath has enabled you to breathe in more easily. If you feel there is more of an opening and spreading, more of an upliftment on the inhalation, then it means that the heart can lift more, give you more joy; it can energize you. So persevere.

There are fun ways of helping this, such as jumping over waves, quite high waves (not frightening ones though), in the sea. If you can actually leap up and jump over the waves, going with the sea, it is the best thing of all; but even imagining yourself doing so would help. Or imagine yourself going up and up and up on a big dipper at the fair—and then suddenly swooping down. The wave pictures in the book are included because to imagine your a looking at these waves helps you to breathe in, to take life in, to open yourself to life.

CHAPTER 2
Using All the Lungs

Few if any people breathe out and empty their lungs sufficiently. Far too many breathe only with the top of their lungs, retaining in the lower parts of the lungs an accumulation of stale and poisonous air. This is a bad habit which may continue for a whole lifetime. Learn to breathe deeply, and to exhale fully, but this will not become a habit without considerable application. You must also learn to breathe slowly, quietly, harmoniously, gradually drawing in the breath deeper and deeper until you fill and empty the lower part of the lungs, expanding the ribs fully as you inhale.

Here is an exercise for you: having first cleaned the nostrils, stand if possible before an open window. As you inhale each breath aspire to God, feel that God is entering into you. Then, as you exhale, send out your blessing upon all life. This inbreathing will cause the spiritual sunlight to fill and illumine you, and register on a chakra or psychic centre situated at the brow. From that centre you can mentally direct the light to the heart centre in order to bring spiritual sunlight to the seed atom which rests in the human heart. Do this each day if you can, and for as long as you like, but without strain.

White Eagle, SPIRITUAL UNFOLDMENT I *(Liss, Hants., 1961)*

'OF COURSE I use my lungs to breathe', I hear you say. Yes, but most of us only breathe with the top front part of our lungs, and use only the secondary respiratory muscles that run up the top of the chest and into the neck.

The breath is actually drawn in by creating space in the whole body, so reducing the pressure on the inside of the body compared with that on the outside. When we do this, the breath wants to fill up that space to equalize the pressure.

To create this space, the diaphragms of the pelvic floor and the thoracic cavity need to spread out and down (see Chapter 3 for an account of the diaphragms). The pelvic-floor diaphragm needs to spread so that all the lower abdominal organs relax down and give space for the thoracic diaphragm to spread down and out. This, the diaphragm that we most associate with the breathing, is attached to the ribcage at the sides, to the spine at the back and to the sternum at the front. It is shaped like a parachute and anchored to the spine by the long tendinous crura muscles. The diaphragm, the crura and the intercostal muscles joining the diaphragm to the rib-cage are known as the primary respiratory muscles. The thoracic diaphragm can be partially frozen, held in spasm or tightened by events in our lives that have caused us to withdraw and grip ourselves tightly in the solar plexus area—or simply through living life under the appalling strain that most of the

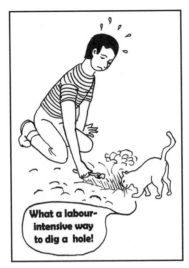

What a labour-intensive way to dig a hole!

time we inflict on ourselves today.

With the diaphragm frozen, we are forced to use only the secondary respiratory muscles in the top chest. This is like the man in the cartoon using a kitchen fork to dig a hole, and is very tiring. We then do not really take the air in fully, but use just the top part of the lungs. The largest part of the lungs is actually in the back of the ribcage. So if we can consciously take the breath into the back body we can free up the diaphragm and gradually bring it back to its full movement.

PRACTICE 1: TO FEEL THE BACK OF THE BODY

LIE FLAT on your back on a firm surface, preferably the floor, although a firm bed can also be helpful. Feel your breath move in and out. See if you can feel the belly fill and then try to feel the spread back into the pelvis and sacrum bone. It takes a while for the breath to deepen naturally, so don't try to force the breath in.

As you inhale again, can you feel the breath spread across the back body—across the back of the pelvis, the back of the lungs and the back of the ribcage? Exhale when you are ready.

See if each time you breathe is a little easier. Is there more opening and spread into the back body? Do you feel this spread coming up from the pelvis, opening across the back ribs, and going right up between the shoulderblades? Can you feel the opening out, just as your body tells you to exhale again?

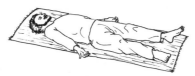

How much more open are you, relaxing into the back of your body as you breathe?

Feeling the breath in the back will help you handle all sorts of situations in life. If you are confronted by an angry person, or you notice an angry response in yourself, or you are facing something which makes you anxious, then see if you can breathe and open into the back of the body. If you do this, you will not feel your chest and pelvis pushed forward and up to confront the person or event, but rather will work from a more relaxed, open space. Your back will then be broader for you to take all life has to offer you. You will be in charge.

From lying, gently roll onto one side and then the other to come up to a sitting position.

Once you have been able to feel the breath in the back of your body while you are lying down, you can then feel it sitting (where a friend can help by putting their hands on your back ribs, see page 20), and then standing—and ultimately in any situation in life. As you breathe more in the back of the body you will feel the diaphragms (see p. 25) opening and spreading all the time.

In every situation your life brings, take a moment to think of your breath. Feel the spreading back and the opening out that the breath can give to your body. From this, a relaxing, releasing and opening of the mind naturally follows: one that enables your perceptions to expand. No longer are you closed in on the situation. Instead, you get a wider view of your life and all that is happening for you.

PRACTICE 2 : TO ENCOURAGE USE OF THE WHOLE LUNGS

ONCE we can consciously breathe into the back of the ribcage, we can take things further. The best way to proceed is to lie down again on a firm surface so that you can feel the back of your body, or alternatively—if you prefer standing or sitting—to have someone put their hands on the back ribs as you breathe into them. This will help you feel what you are doing.

Consciously bring the gaze of your eyes down into your body. Imagine that you can see right through your body to the sacrum, the back ribs, even the shoulderblade area. Feel the breath filling into the back body. Feel the sacrum spreading, as though the bones of this area are spreading on the firmness of the earth underneath you. Feel the back ribs opening and spreading as you inhale.

Gently exhale, whenever you are ready, and feel the movement of the breath into the sacrum, the back ribs and the shoulderblades. It will be even more after a few breaths. The upper back spreads down between the shoulderblades as you exhale. Feel the diaphragm where it attaches to the lumbar spine and the side ribs. Feel where you can open and spread. As you inhale, the diaphragm spreads out and down, giving that broadening of the back; and as you exhale, you may feel the diaphragm rise up as a dome. You may feel the side ribs contract, for all the lower ribs come in to let the breath go out.

It helps also to breathe into one side, to feel the breath spread into first the left side of the pelvis, the left sacrum, the left ribs, the left shoulderblades. This way, you have more emphasis on the opening from the spine out to the left. Do this for a few breaths, and when you have done that, and after an exhalation, change your awareness to the right side. Now feel the *prana*, the life-force, filling into the right sacrum, the right back ribs, the right shoulderblade. Exhale so that you spread from the centre of the spine to the right and down.

When you have done that for a few breaths, come back to breathing through the centre and feel as though you have got even more breadth into the back body now. Feel it from the spine and extending through the back ribs and to the shoulderblades. See if there is greater movement and opening there: maybe you can even feel the air in the back where most of the lung area is. The very pores in the skin of the back body open more.

Do this for five to ten minutes as your relaxation, and then roll onto your side and sit for a few minutes. See if you can feel that same awareness while you are sitting. You can sit against the wall, or you can even sit against another person (see p. 12), because then you can feel them breathing as well. You can breathe into one another.

When you have sat for as long as you want to, see if you can feel that same awareness of breathing into the back body standing. Little by little, take that awareness into the whole of your life. It's very helpful consciously to practise this in situations in your life where you may feel angry or anxious.

Maybe you are nervous about an interview. Maybe there is something you particularly want to say or are not sure how to say it. Someone else may be angry and speaking to you in a way that you don't find easy to take. In any such situation, consciously take your breath into the back of the body. Literally broaden your back to take whatever the world has for you there. The situation is there for you to understand, to experience, not to retract from.

Before you respond, take a few breaths into the back of your body and you may feel your response will be less of a knee-jerk one. It does not have to be the reaction which has come from past experience with the person or from your patterning. Instead, it can be a response that is open, aware—even, in a way, vulnerable, for by broadening your back you are making yourself stronger and actually taking what life has to give you rather than pushing it away. If the back of the body is broad and strong, then the front of the body can soften and relax. It actually relaxes into the back of the body. So what you have—instead of a cramped, tense reaction to events—is a conscious, contained vulnerability (a sensitivity to what others are feeling), which comes from a more aware space in yourself.

Because you are fully conscious of how you are responding, you are neither making yourself over-vulnerable, nor are you closing down. Symbolically, the back of the body is the strong part, connected with the earth and entrenched in matter, while the front is the soft part of the body and has this capacity to be open to whatever events in life come to us. You are keeping a balance between the back and the front. You are dealing not just with the impact of the events but with your response to them.

It takes some experience to be able to do this all the time, so don't expect the practice to solve everything in your life immediately. Yet through doing it, maybe daily, initially lying on your back, then sitting and standing, you will see what a difference it makes. See if breathing into the back body gives you a broader perception, a wider encompassing of whatever is going on around you.

MUDRAS

When all the knots of the heart are broken, then the mortal becomes immortal. Katha Upanishad 6.15

Mudra means gesture or attitude, while *hasta* means hand. Hand gestures express but also channel the energy of the body. A handshake was originally to show that neither person had a weapon in their hands, and is more to do with the ego self. The gesture known as *namaste* in Sanskrit (*anjali* in Pali) placing the hands together over the heart and bowing towards one another—is a greeting from the heart indicating we are in harmony with one another. *Mudras* are used in yoga to focus awareness in a certain area.

The subtle or breath body (in Sanskrit the *prana maya kosa*) connects mind to prana, life-force. *Maya* means the layer of illusion that is the physical world, and *kosa*, a veil or sheath. Throughout this subtle body there are channels of energy known in Sanskrit as *nadis*. These are like paths, rivers, radio waves and all the ways in which energy is channelled through earth and space. Acupuncture, shiatsu and reflexology rely on these energy channels to heal the physical body (the *ana maya kosa*: *ana* translates as food). In yoga *asana* and *pranayama* we move and clear the energy in these channels.

The main *nadi* that runs through the body is the *chitta nadi*. *Chitta* is the heart-consciousness (in Buddhist teaching), or the higher consciousness, the collective aspects of the mind that have the potential to connect to and blend into the Self (*Atman* or *Purusha*), the Divine in us. The root 'chit' means to be aware, so a clear flow in this *nadi* brings awareness within us and around us. The main channel for the *chitta* energy is the *susumna* that runs through the spinal column and corresponds to the central spinal cord in the physical body. Hence the importance of a lengthened, strong spine.

Mudras are employed in *asana*, *pranayama* and meditation to contain and focus this energy. For example, *chin mudra* (where the tip of the index finger is reined in initially to the first thumb-joint and then to the root of the thumb), brings an opening at the level of the thoracic and throat diaphragms, while *gyana mudra* (where the tip of the index finger touches the tip of the thumb) connects to the pelvic diaphragm.

PRACTICE 3 : TO MOVE THE DIAPHRAGMS USING *CHIN* AND *GYANA MUDRA*—ATTITUDE OR GESTURE OF CONSCIOUSNESS

SIT in any posture that is comfortable to you, but make sure your spine is lengthened and that you feel the base spreading and the heart open. Rest the backs of the hands on the thighs, and open all your fingers out to stretch them. Then bring the tip of the index finger to touch the tip of the thumb on each hand (middle drawing). This is known in yoga as *gyana mudra*.

Be aware now of your breath moving through your body. Does your awareness come right down across the base to feel the spread of the pelvic-floor diaphragm as you inhale? Is there a gentle doming in and up, creating a *bandha* (a containing of the prana to move it up, see p. 26) across the base, the *muladhara chakra* or *mula bandha*?

It may take several breaths to become aware of this movement or even to enable the movement. Or it may take weeks, years of practice—I realize and feel more day by day after thirty-three years of practice—so don't give up on it easily! When you have felt this movement of the pelvic diaphragm, rein the index finger (representing the *ahamkar*, the ego, translated as the awareness of the existence of 'I') in to touch the first joint of the thumb, nearest the nail (right-hand diagram).

Does that make a difference to your awareness of your breath moving through your body? Can you feel the opening of the thoracic diaphragm more now, at the level of the solar plexus, spreading down and out as you inhale, doming in and up as you exhale?

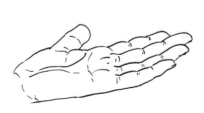
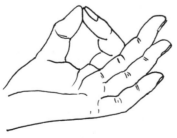
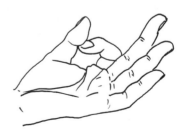

Again, stay with your breath as long as your mind is able. This may feel different with each time of practice.

Now rein the index finger in more to touch the root of the thumb. Where does that bring your awareness now? Is it across the base of the throat, so that you feel the movement of the vocal diaphragm, doming up as you inhale, flattening down as you exhale?

All these diaphragms increase the space in the chest to open the lungs to the air, *prana*, then decrease the space to let the breath go out. The hand-position with the index finger to the first and second joint of the thumb is known as *chin mudra*. *Chin* means 'attitude of consciousness', while *gyana* means 'attitude of knowledge'. The latter connects to *mula bandha*

(*bandhas* are explained on page 26) at the level of the base of the spine and so encourages the movement of the pelvic-floor diaphragm. In *chin mudra*, there is more opening higher up the body in the thoracic and throat diaphragms.

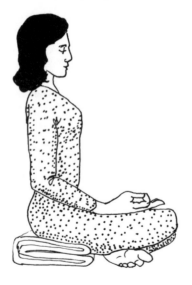

These mudras therefore connect mind and body, using the breath as a conscious connection: they are a step towards the creation of a union of the whole self. It is important, though, not to force the practice of these *mudras*, and not to just put the fingers into the position automatically. Rather, let them evolve naturally out of your awareness of your breath as you sit, so you stay with that conscious connection. Let the mind go with the breath moving through the body: you do not want the mind to be dictating where the fingers go, but rather the other way round.

The three phases of *chin mudra*, including *gyana mudra*, can be practised one after another. Then feel how you can go on to breathe full breaths, with the whole of the body involved in the process.

CHAPTER 3
The Diaphragms of the Body

DIAPHRAGMS are layers of strong, flat, tendinous muscle which can broaden and open out. There are three main ones in the body. The lowest is positioned across the base—almost literally to stop the guts falling out. The next is beneath the ribs, and stops the lungs and heart falling into the abdominal organs. The uppermost is positioned across the throat to contain the voice-box.

To feel the three diaphragms, use a very simple breathing exercise. Standing where you can breathe in fresh air, let the arms open to the side as you inhale (left-hand diagram). Exhale when you are ready. This initial opening of the arms will move the pelvic diaphragm. As the breath comes in again, spread the arms out more to shoulder level (central diagram),

and you will feel the ribs spread, thus opening the thoracic diaphragm. Exhale, and let your arms come up over your head. When you inhale again with the arms over your head (right-hand diagram), you will feel the throat open. Exhale, bring the palms together and down through the front of the

body and back down to the base. Repeat this breath, known as the Tree of Light, at least twice more to feel the opening it brings.

The base diaphragm, known as the pelvic floor, is in the same region as the perineum. This is the

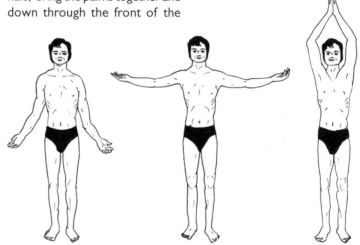

area across the base from the pubic bone to the tail bone and across to each buttock bone. It spreads down and out with the inhalation to make more space in the lower abdomen or belly. In turn, that encourages the thoracic diaphragm (attached to the ribcage at the sides, the lumbar spine at the back, and the breastbone at the front) to open down and out like an arc. A greater volume of space is created in the chest area. This reduces the pressure there, so that the air rushes in. The diaphragm at the base of the throat is associated with the voice box. When you inhale, it domes up and this too creates more space in the chest cavity, allowing the breath to come in.

The three diaphragms need to work together to permit a full inhalation. On the exhalation, the two lower diaphragms (across the base and across the ribcage) dome up. The diaphragm in the throat flattens down to reduce the space or volume in the chest cavity. Thus the pressure of the air becomes greater and so it goes out. This mechanical action of the diaphragm is what generates the movement of the breath, in and out. On the inbreath, it can feel as though the breath is going right down into the belly. What is actually happening is that the two lower diaphragms are doming down and creating more space for the lungs to expand into, so the breath fills the full enclosed space of the lungs.

At the same time there is cellular breathing—where all the cells of the skin, but also all the cells of the body pulsate. They open with the inhalation and soften with the exhalation.

BANDHAS

What in yoga are known as bandhas are at the level of the diaphragms but in the subtle body (prana maya kosa). The word bandha otherwise means a lock—not the lock which needs a key, keeping some things in and others out, but more the lock of a canal which contains moving water within a certain area. Thus a bandha contains prana within an area of the body. They are shaped like gentle domes.

The mula bandha, around the base of the spine (more properly, around the base chakra, muladhara chakra), gently domes on the inhalation, creating a movement of pranic energy. This movement of prana continues of the exhalation, but there is a movement down and out of apana, the outward-moving energy.

The uddiyana bandha, at the level of the solar plexus, creates an arc to take the prana into the heart area, and focus the consciousness—chitta—in the heart. The jalandhara bandha creates a dome in the throat to release the head energy down to the heart.

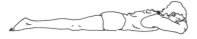

FEELING YOUR BREATH, LYING ON YOUR FRONT

LIE face down, flat on the floor and easing your hips into the ground. Rock them a little from side to side to relax them down. Rest your forehead on your hands and ease your elbows out, so that you are comfortable. Now bring your awareness down so that you feel the movement of your tummy against the floor as you breathe in and out. You can do this on a bed but you actually feel it more on the firmness of the floor.

Feel how the breath spreads—the movement all around the tummy, all around the pelvis—and feel the movement there as you in-hale and exhale. This is a way of developing an awareness of how the breath movement starts right in the base diaphragm. You can feel it in the pelvis, across the peri-neum, which spreads right across the base from the anus through to the vaginal wall in a woman and the scrotum in a man.

As you gradually become aware of the breath movement, you may find that it doesn't always move as easily into one side of the pelvis as the other. One side may feel more open to the breath than the other. If it feels as though it is not moving so easily on one side, then turn your head to that side and rest your opposite cheekbone on your hands. Does that make a differ-ence? Does that encourage the *prana* to move better and fill the lower body more on that side? As you breathe, first feel the move-ment deep into the pelvis and then up into the ribcage, up into the top chest. With your head on one side, does it feel as though there is more opening there?

If it does, then after a few breaths that way, bring your head back to the centre. Now, does that movement of the breath into that side stay with you when the head is in the centre? Whether there is really an even spread or if it is just more even than it was before, now turn your head to the other side.

Does that encourage the breath to move deep into the lungs on that side and open into the pelvis, into the ribcage, into the chest? Can you feel a similar effect when you exhale? Stay with this for a few breaths, for half a dozen maybe. Then bring your head back to the centre and see if it has made a dif-ference this way round. See if you now have more balance between the two sides of the body.

Next, go back simply to feeling the breath movement, deep in the belly, right from the pubic bone up to the top of the pelvis. Then when you are ready to move, bring your hands back by your ribs, and take your knees firmly into the ground, to lift your hips. Spread the sacrum as you inhale.

Bring your buttocks back onto your heels, resting your brow on

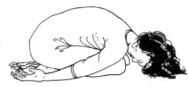

the ground in front of your knees. This is known in yoga as child pose, *balasana*, illustrated above (it is also sometimes called *pindasana*, mouse pose). At this point, inhaling, you can really feel the movement of the belly and the ribcage,

spreading onto the thighs. Be aware of how much movement there is in the body to enable the breath to come. Then discover what happens to the ribs and the belly as the breath goes out. If you have the brow resting down on the ground this relaxes and releases the head, while also making a real connection between the head, and brings the awareness into the body through the breath.

CHAPTER 4
Sound

OM,
The imperishable sound,
   is the seed of all that exists.
The past, the present, the future,
   —all are but the unfolding of OM.
And, whatever transcends the three realms of
   time,
that indeed is the flowering of OM.

This whole creation is ultimately Brahman.
And the self,
   this also is Brahman.

This pure self has four quarters:

The first is the waking state,
   experience of the reality common to everyone,
The attention faces outwards,
   enjoying the world in all its variety.

The second is experience of subjective worlds,
   such as in dreaming.
Here the attention dwells within,
   charmed by the mind's subtler creations.

The third is deep sleep,
   the mind rests, with awareness suspended.
This state beyond duality,
   —from which the waves of thinking emerge,
   is enjoyed by the enlightened as an ocean of
   silence and bliss.

The fourth, say the wise, is the pure Self alone.
Dwelling in the heart of all,
   it is the lord of all,
   the seer of all,
   the source and goal of all.

It is not outer awareness,
It is not inner awareness,
Nor is it a suspension of awareness.
It is not knowing,

It is not unknowing,
Nor is it knowingness itself.
It can neither be seen nor understood,
It cannot be given boundaries.
It is ineffable and beyond thought.
It is indefinable.
It is known only through becoming it.
It is the end of all activity,
    silent and unchanging,
    the supreme good,
    one without a second.
It is the real Self.
It, above all, should be known.

This pure Self and OM are as one;
    and the different quarters of the Self
    correspond to OM and its sounds, A-U-M.

Experience of the outer world corresponds to A,
    the first sound.
This initiates action and achievement.
Whoever awakens to this acts in freedom and
    achieves success.

Experience of the inner world corresponds to U,
    the second sound.
This initiates upholding and unification.
Whoever awakens to this upholds the tradition
    of knowledge and unifies the diversities of life
Everything that comes along speaks to him of
    Brahman.

The state of dreamless sleep corresponds to M,
    the third sound.
This initiates measurement and merging.
Whoever awakens to this merges with the world
    and has the measure of all things.

The pure Self alone,
    that which is indivisible,
    which cannot be described,
    the supreme good,
    the one without a second,
That corresponds to the wholeness of OM.
Whoever awakens to that becomes the Self.

Mandukya Upanishad,
translated by Alistair Shearer and Peter Russell,
Harper & Row, New York, 1978

THE BREATH AND SOUND

ONE of the most important ways of breathing out is in making sound. This can be the sound we make speaking, but also singing, sounding individual notes, or chanting.

The expression of the OM as set out in the Upanishads on the previous pages is a way of sounding what is deep within us and has been there since the beginning of creation. The OM is an expression of creation itself: what brought us into being; a remembering of the Big Bang, if you like. As St John tells us, 'In the beginning was the Word'.

The OM evolves out of the three sounds 'A' (ah), 'U' (oo) and 'M', creating AUM. Sounded together, they blend to 'OM'. If we want to sound the AUM, the first sound 'A' is the expression of our self moving outwards from the centre. It is our expressing of our-

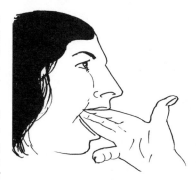

selves in the outer world. Through 'A' we are present in our everyday world of interaction, speaking, acting. It is good to practise a few 'A's at first. If you want to do this, find yourself a quiet place where you won't be overheard, or choose the company of others who want to join together with you and express that outward moving.

One way to develop the 'A' sound is by having the mouth very open. The teacher John-David Biggs advises his students to put

three fingers in between the teeth in order to get the mouth wide enough to get that deep expression of the A to come out. It comes from deep in the self, deep in the belly, 'AAAAAA'. (There is a CD on chanting by John-David called THE PERFECT PRAYER. For details, see p. 64.) If you can make the sound from this deep level, you can really feel how it initiates a moving outwards in action, in being able to act on our own truth.

When we come to the 'U' vowel, which is sounded as 'oo', the tongue wants to be in the middle of the mouth. The teeth remain open, but are more closed than in making the 'A' sound. The sense of 'UUUUUU' may then come clearly: it is something more inner, more an expression of how we are inwardly.

Now the 'MMMMMM' emerges, a developed hum, suspending all

other sound. If we practise it with the teeth a little open, the lips closed, the tongue again in the centre of the mouth, then that sense of the 'M' can take us to a very quiet, deep still place.

I have found it is helpful to practise each sound several times to get the sense of them all individually, and then join them together in the AUM sound. The unified chant then expresses the pure self, dwelling in the heart of all and then the joined vowels, which make an 'oohh', to me is the joining together of our outer expression and inner expression of ourselves. In this sound we can outwardly express who we really are, how we really are. When the 'A', 'U' and 'M' come together, the past, present and future are all joining in one in the flowering of the OM.

Chanting the OM requires some practice and can be done in many different ways. The way to do it can be experimented with, using short sounds or long sounds. However, it has more power when sounded clearly and strongly: it is uplifting then both for the one who sounds it and for anyone listening.

We need a sense of how all three diaphragms work to produce sound well: not only the diaphragm

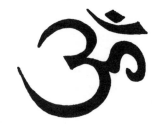

in the throat, connected to the voice box, but the diaphragms in the base and in the thoracic cavity. Those diaphragms really need to move if the expression of the sound is to be clear and outgoing.

There are many other sounds, many other mantras that can be chanted. If you want to pursue this way of developing the breath, you need to find out for yourself what feels most appropriate and helpful for you. You may also discover what best expresses how you are at any one time. For instance, when you are feeling angry there may be some particular sound which will usefully express and hold that anger.

Sometimes when we meditate there actually needs to be some tears, some sobbing, which can be helped by chanting. Meditation can evoke all sorts of things, and chanting may be a controlled vocal expression of them. Yoga students may also find that chanting helps in the postures. For instance, we can open ourselves more into back bends by emitting a sharp clear sound as we go into them. There are mantras which express the chakras, and sometimes if we feel an opening of the chakra there is a sound that expresses that.

Equally, it may feel better for you

to sound 'amen' or 'alleluia' rather than the OM. I remember a conversation I had with a Hindu man in India who said that India has the OM and Christianity has the Amen. That is a link between them, he said: the expression in sound of the inner being. What we are sounding may be an expression of our own personal history, or it may be an expression of the whole consciousness of humanity from the very beginning.

PRACTICE : MOVEMENT OF THE SPINE WITH THE MOVEMENT OF THE BREATH

LIE down on your back, with your knees bent up, your feet firm on the earth, your arms spread out to the side (see 'Preparation', page 11), so that the hips and the chest feel spread into the ground at the back, and opened out at the front. Bring your awareness right down through the length of your body and out across the breadth of your body. Be aware of the breath moving in; be aware of the spread of the pelvic floor as the breath comes in, and remain aware of it as it goes out.

Feel the position of the coccyx (the base of the spine) at the level of the pelvic floor. As you inhale, can you feel that subtle lengthening-down of the base of the spine? Can you feel how the whole spine lengthens with that movement down and away towards the feet,

down towards the ground? It is as though the whole spine undoes and eases out with the inhalation.

Now, on the exhalation, feel the base of the spine moving slightly up. Then as you inhale, again feel that lengthening down, which allows the lumbar spine to come into its natural arch and the breastbone to spread and open out. As you exhale, feel how the upper back spreads down, the lumbar area spreads back and down, and the tailbone rolls up.

Inhaling again, can you feel, with that rolling down of the tailbone, that the bottom of the sacrum spreads out and down more into the ground, while the top of the pelvis tilts slightly up and the breastbone fills? As you exhale, it is the reverse of that: the upper back spreads down and the top of

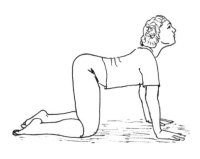
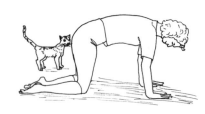

the pelvis and the top of the sacrum also spread down. The lumbar spine flattens out, and the tailbone rolls up.

The whole rhythm of your breath thus massages and moves the whole spine and the whole of the inner body, the vital organs, with it. So as you go with the spine in this way, the belly softens and relaxes, the throat relaxes back and the whole body broadens and opens. The back body lengthens and strengthens, the front body softens and opens.

This is actually what they are intended to do—not to remain tight and motionless. For full anatomical explanations and drawings see Donna Farhi, THE BREATHING BOOK (details, p. 64).

If it is difficult to feel, lying on your back, all that I have asked you to feel, then you could come onto all fours like a cat and feel the very subtle beginning movement of what in yoga is known as the cat pose (*bindalasana*). Imagine the tailbone lengthening up and away, just like a cat's tail does. As you inhale, and feel this, move the whole spine, giving the slight arch of the lumbar spine and the movement forward of the breastbone shown in the drawing. As you exhale, feel the back flatten and broaden, and spread up.

CHAPTER 5
Breathing and Emotion: Anger and Calm

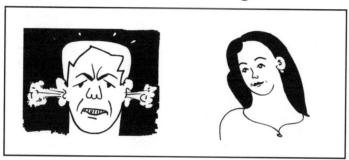

WHAT goes on in your breathing when you are angry and feel under strain? Does it feel held? Does it feel as though you are bursting to breathe but unable to because you are just so wound up and angry? What would be the effect of a little bit of gentle inhalation and exhalation when you feel angry?

In each of Chapters 5 to 8, we shall be dealing with specific emotions—anger, despair, fear, grief—with breathing practices to help.

DEALING WITH FEELINGS OF ANGER OR RESENTMENT, OR WHEN WANTING TO YELL OR SWEAR AT SOMEONE

When they are angry, people tend to puff out their cheeks and push the breath out as a sort of release. This reaction is one that people demonstrate when they are trying to gather themselves. When you too feel angry, it's helpful con-

sciously to do the same, or even consciously to make a sound as you force the breath out: *ahhhhh!* or *phhhhh!* If you are confronted with a situation that makes you angry, then rather than yelling or swearing, try to have a sense of really exhaling the sound. Next, take the breath into the back body, as we have now learnt to do. If you feel you need to, do it again and maybe again. Don't worry if people think you are strange: it's

35

easier for them than yelling at them, isn't it?

The alternative may be a knee-jerk reaction. You may recall times in your life about which you think, 'Why did I say that? Why did I react like that? Where did it come from? It doesn't feel like me to say that'. These hasty reactions tend to arise from our past patterning. They are part of how we have learned to defend ourselves. Although they have given us that defence, they don't actually serve us in relationships, because they antagonize the other person.

If we are wanting to start anew in relationships and to let go of past patterning, what we want to be able to do is train ourselves in how to respond. A response is a very different thing from a reaction. We call our reactions knee-jerks because they are out of our control. The heartfelt response, perhaps from greater wisdom, can be instantaneous too, yet often the knee-jerk reaction gets in first and so comes in the way of that.

Above all, if we take a moment to breathe, and remember to fill the back body; if we exhale and make a sigh as we do, then we are more likely to give a heart response, one which has let go of past patterning. If we want to be able to open our hearts in response to one another, the breathing is the key. While the breath is uncontrolled, all of the patterning that we have will be reflected in how we inhale and exhale. As we become aware of how we breathe, when we breathe and where we breathe in our bodies, control of the whole pattern of how we react also becomes possible.

PRACTICE 1

EVEN if we don't feel angry at the moment, most of us can remember a situation when we did. For this practice, call up from your memory a situation where you felt angry. Explore the feeling for a moment. Alternatively, see in your imagination someone whom you felt or feel angry with. See that person in front of you. See what it is about them, about what they are saying, that makes you angry; see what it is that stirs you up, that you don't want to hear, that you don't want to know. Maybe what you feel is that you want to retaliate in some way.

Then see what happens to your breath the moment you experience that anger. Is it held in? Are you holding the diaphragm tight? Are you stiffening your shoulders and tightening your throat? Have you gritted your jaw and tightened your tongue? How does your body feel? How does the breath feel, and how does the breath reflect that feeling in the body?

The movement of the breath and the level of tension or relaxation in the body are dependent on one another. In order to tighten the body up, you have to hold your breath, and in order to hold your breath, you have to tighten your body up: tighten your diaphragm, tighten your throat, tighten even your anus and along the perineum. Hold your breath. Can you feel this tightening in the different areas of the body?

Now see what happens if you consciously breathe right down into the belly. Instead of the tightening you have been feeling, release the diaphragms in the base and the thoracic cavity. Let the breath fill into them, and then gently let yourself exhale again. There might need to be a sound on the exhalation fully to release the tension. This may take a few breaths. It might actually take a few weeks, even a few years of practice at this, to discover how you can change your breath-pattern: how you can learn to breath when you have otherwise not been breathing, how you can exhale when before your breath was held.

If at least in the imagined situation you are able to manage some release of your breath, what happens to what you are feeling? Try and be more thoughtful for a moment. Try and remember the difference between 'react' and 'respond'. Reactions are out of our control, but responses can be from the heart, in openness and clarity.

In a situation that feels unjust to us, are we strong enough to speak our truth? Are we able to do it from a clear, open, strong space: strong in the back body, rather than from an out-of-control reaction?

Leaving the other behind, create a situation or a theme or a feeling in your body that makes you feel calm and at peace with yourself and the world around you. This may be a view of the countryside, of a still lake, of a mountain. Get this vision in your mind or actually go and sit looking at a view you find peaceful. You may have a place you know where you feel at one with nature, at ease in yourself. See what happens now to the feelings you may have had, of anger and frustration.

As they calm down, what happens to your breathing? Has it changed because you have put yourself in a situation that calms you; does your breathing reflect the beautiful place you have put yourself in, either in imagination or in fact? Or is it that the breathing helps to create that calm? Can you bring the two together: the awareness of the breath and the calming place?

Try and be aware of how your breath is now, so that if you are somewhere where you can't be in an outwardly peaceful situation, you create that awareness instead by your breath. You never know when you may be in a situation

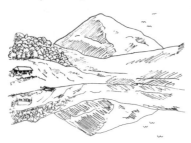

where you cannot get to a quiet or peaceful spot—where you may get 'trapped in the marketplace', as it were. You need always to be able to find that peace and quiet within yourself. When, outwardly, you are stuck in a situation not of your own choosing, can you be aware, can you breathe, can you open, can you stay calm?

To do so obviously takes a great deal of perseverance and practice, but who knows when any of us will be in a situation, temporary or long-term, that we can't get out of? Our mind has an enormous capacity to create calmness and peace in its awareness. That can be done through the breath and is totally reflected in the breath. You will gradually recognize this as you practise awareness of the breath.

BALANCING ENERGY IN THE BODY : NADI SODHANA WITH PADMA HASTA MUDRA (ALTERNATE NOSTRIL BREATHING WITH HAND GESTURE)

> *Pingala is the dynamic male principle and ida the passive female principle. The left brain hemisphere operates on the same principle as pingala. It processes information logically, sequentially, and functions according to time sequence. The right hemisphere is concerned with intuition, mental creativity and orientation in space. When both nostrils operate simultaneously the energy is being transferred from one hemisphere to the other. It passes through a thin sheet of membrane between the two hemispheres called the corpus callosum. At this time the whole brain can function and perception will not be limited to one mode of processing.*
>
> *Hatha Yoga Pradipika*, trans. Swami Saraswati

THE practice of *nadi sodhana*, alternate nostril breathing, along with what translates as the Lotus Hand Mudra (illustrated in the right hand in the drawing, right), has the effect of calming the whole system down. It soothes and settles the mind, and can relieve headaches and stress. The aim in doing it is to balance the body, mind and emotions, and to tone the internal organs; it is said to enable the intestines to work more efficiently.

It is most effective to do it sit-

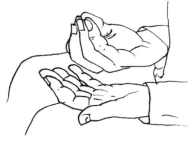

ting with the spine upright (see page 11). This and the *hasta mudra* create more opening in the body for the breath to come in.

Doing *nadi sodhana* with *padma*

hasta mudra enables one side of the body at a time to open to the breath. Usually, in ordinary breathing, one nostril is more open than the other. You can feel this by becoming aware of your breaths over a period of time: they can vary from hour to hour and throughout different times of the day. You may also develop a sense of the *nadis* (see p. 22).

The *pingala nadi* is the channel for the dynamic outgoing, active male principle, while the *ida nadi* carries the more inner, nurturing, female principle. These two nadis spiral around the *susumna nadi*, that travels the length of the spine. When the breath flows more through the left nostril, *ida* is more active, and when the breath flows through the right nostril *pingala* is more active. A direct link is established here between the *ana maya kosa* (the physical body) and the *prana maya kosa* (the breath or subtle body). By virtue of this, this *pranayama* brings balance to the whole system.

By balancing the breath in the two nostrils, *nadi sodhana* also balances the two hemispheres of the brain. This may give a clue as to why it is so helpful to practise it regularly.

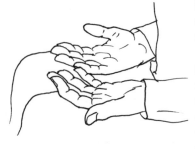

NADI SODHANA

SIT cross-legged or in *virasana* (with feet to the side) or on a chair in such a way that the spine is lengthened and the chest opened. Place the back of the hands on your thighs, just above your knees, palms facing the ceiling, so that your shoulders and elbows drop down and the thoracic diaphragm spreads. Bring your awareness to your breath for a several inhalations and exhalations until it deepens and evens out and the mind can begin to settle. Then open all the fingers out on both hands like the petals of a flower opening out wide to the sun (shown in the drawing, left).

Notice the difference that makes to the way the breath moves through your body. The palm of the hand is itself a *chakra* (an energy centre), so feel the opening there that sympathetically opens the whole body out to the incoming breath.

After a few breaths, bring the fingers and thumbs together on both hands, the fingertips pointing upwards to the sky, so that each finger touches the thumb. It is as though the petals of the flower are closing in. This position reminds me of a lotus or a tulip. In both flowers, the petals go in and up when they close. This is the lotus hand gesture, *padma hasta mudra*, shown in the right hand of the drawing on page 39.

Notice what happens to the breath now. How does the diaphragm move? After a few breaths,

40

open wide the fingers on the left hand only. Let the breath come in, feeling if it comes more into the left side, filling the pelvis, rib cage, left nostril, even the left hemisphere of the brain. Breathe out, feeling if the breath goes out more through the left side. Repeat this on the left side for several breaths.

Then, at the end of an exhalation, close the fingers of the left hand, and open the ones on the right hand. Feel now if the breath comes more through the whole of the right side, even as though it goes through the palm of the hand and goes out through the right side. Continue this for a few breaths.

At the end of an exhalation, close the fingers on the right hand; take a few easy breaths through both nostrils, aware of how the breath feels in the body now. When you feel ready, open the fingers on the left side and let the breath fill the left side, till the top of the inhalation. Then close the fingers on the left hand, open the fingers on the right hand, and exhale through the right nostril and side. Keep the fingers open, inhale through the right side; and this time at the top of the inhalation, close the fingers on the right side, open the fingers on the left side, and exhale through the left nostril. Continue this movement from side to side, changing the fingers at the top of each breath until you feel ready to rest, letting your fingers open into a natural relaxed *mudra* (i.e., an ordinary open-handed gesture) and let the breath gently come in through both sides.

Feel how open the body is now, how much the breath can fill the body, then breathe out completely.

CHAPTER SIX
Breathing and Emotion: Depression and Happiness

SOMETIMES, inevitably, we feel despairing or depressed. This can be anything from a passing mood or phase to a bout of clinical depression. Whatever the causes of

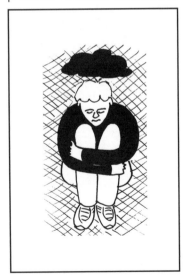

the depression, and whether they are recent or way back, the body closes in on itself, the shoulders hunch, and the heart area tends to be very 'held': closed in. So the breath becomes shallow and we breathe very little. Sometimes we do not breathe much at all. A few opening yoga postures would help here, if you are trained in yoga. They may produce tears—which would, if so, be healing. Alternatively, they might produce feelings of hurt or anger. If they do, stay with these feelings, let them be, and go into a gentle *ujjayi pranayama,* the breathing practice given on p. 45. Otherwise, follow the practice set out opposite.

In today's quick-satisfaction society, we can feel that happiness is something that can be bought, or

for which we are dependent on someone else. We think of it coming to us by chance and circumstance. In yogic and Buddhist paths it is considered that a state of happiness or contentment (*santosa* in Sanskrit) needs to be cultivated and worked at. One way is through postures, breathing and medita-

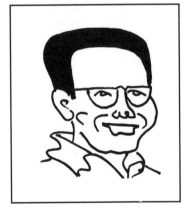

tion, so that we gradually change our outlook on life to one of gratitude and appreciation. Our joy then is in everyday awareness of life.

This may be difficult to conceive of in cases of severe depression and does need some continued practice, but the next two practices really move your energy, and so begin to make this possible.

PRACTICE I

THIS time, sit down or even remain standing . Don't lie down, as it's a bit too relaxing for this exercise! Standing or sitting, we are more open when we summon up the sort of situation we are going to recreate in our awareness. Upright, we are more likely to notice what happens to our breath. Now visualize a situation in your mind where you feel very down, very despairing. Recollect times when you have felt that life is too much, when you've felt unable to cope, or just that your life was getting you down. Are you now aware of what your breathing is like in this situation?

Develop the image by seeing any people who are involved in the situation. Recreate in imagination the location of the situation. See what you might be wearing, what the other person might be wearing, anything that will help to bring

it back. Imagine what you might be feeling and almost invoke the feeling itself; and then say to yourself, 'What is happening to my breath now?'.

You may even like to compare it to a different but similar situation to see what the difference is in what happens to your breath. Take notice of that.

Now, 'What happens if I consciously take my awareness further down into my own being, more into the back of my body? How does my breathing change?'. Notice that too, and carry on for a few more breaths. Notice how the situation feels now. Has anything changed, has your perception of the situation changed?

A full change in the situation may take some practice. We rarely break these long-held habits overnight. I can say from experience that is possible to do so quite suddenly, but this is exceptional. Sometimes, if the change does come dramatically, things later tend to revert, and then we need to be aware of what's happened and stay with the feelings we have, working on them a little bit more.

After noticing what happens with depression, create a situation which makes you feel happy, one that lifts you up and encourages you. See that situation, see what is happening there. Create in your imagination the circumstances around it, the people who might be involved, where you are at the time. Notice how you are feeling, how your mood has changed, and then notice how your breath is in that situation.

What is the difference now from the situation you've just experi-

> *Gaining insight into our own negativity is a lifelong task and one which is capable of almost infinite refinement … but unless we undertake it we will be unable to see where to make the necessary changes in our lives.*
> Dalai Lama

enced? Are you able to breath more easily? Are you more open in your body? Is your diaphragm moving more? Is the ribcage opening more? Does the breath tend to be deeper? Is it more down in the belly than in the upper chest?

Practise a little bit in discovering how that breathing is. You may even find it useful briefly to go back to the thought 'How was I when I was feeling depressed?'. Momen-

tarily create the situation of feeling depressed, while keeping the breath as it was when you created the joyful situation. With the breath going right into the back body, are you so likely to get depressed?

There is a lifetime of practice here, a lifetime of breaking patterns.

Working with negativity, which is what we are doing here, is the same as working with our breath. The breath is at times very refined and capable of changing and moving, but will give us the ability to see where to make the necessary changes. What the Dalai Lama says in the quotation is very apposite, so be ready to apply some perseverance!

PRACTICE 2 : UJJAYI PRANAYAMA

Ujjayi pranayama is a full yogic *pranayama* that is particularly helpful for feelings of depression, despair, lack of energy: for feelings of inability to get going in the day.

Sit with the support of an exercise ball, or a wall with a blanket, or a chair with a cushion, to give the spine an initial easing upward. It is important when we feel down to bring the spine as upright as possible. Usually, it tends to curve forward when we feel low or lacking in energy. Therefore start this practice by easing it backwards. This will lift and open out the breastbone.

From that easing up of the back, bring your awareness to the base of the spine and the whole area across the perineum so that it broadens and increases the contact you feel with the earth. This means that when the breath begins its journey in, it is as though it comes up from the earth underneath you. With this awareness, you can even increase that broadening and lengthening of the tailbone down. This will spread the pelvic-floor diaphragm and provide the movement in the whole pelvis area which gives the space needed for the breath to come and fill it. At the same time the *mula bandha* domes up for the *prana* to rise up the body, just as a wave climbs up to its crest.

There is a paradox here, as the movement on the inhalation is physically an expansion out to the sides, and yet there is also the beginning of a climbing up of the inner energy in the spine. Gradually, you will become aware that this inner lengthening, up through the spine, continues with the exhalation. It is precisely this that shifts the whole energy of body and mind. As you go on with the inhalation and exhalation, feel the expansion outwards comes up and includes the whole chest, back, sides and front, and then at the top of the inhalation (it may take several breaths before you feel this), there is a spread into the back of the throat with a slight drawing sound there.

As you begin to feel this movement into the back of the throat at the top of the inhalation, you may feel that your head wants to come down to bring your chin towards your chest. But keep the rolling up of your breastbone, in order to increase the spreading feeling, right into the back of the throat. There is a very slight pause at the top of the inhalation but it is not a holding at all.

Now exhale. Feel the breath go right back down, deep into the belly, and again feel that rolling of the tailbone slightly forward. Wait, and as the breath finds its way in feel that movement down and back of the tailbone which gives the whole curving-up of the spine, and the accompanying opening-out of the body.

Although the movement into the throat comes naturally, it might take several days, months, even years of practice really to get that feeling. Don't force it in any way. It is curious that the *Hatha Yoga Pradapika* says make this movement very forcefully in the throat so that there is a rasping sound; and yet it says all these movements come naturally with practice. It actually took me years to feel that movement into the back of the throat. To me, it feels much better to let it come naturally than force it, which would possibly cause disturbances in the pattern of the breath. It needs all of the awareness of the breath we can develop before we force this movement at

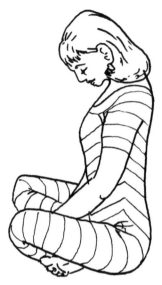

all. Instead, it is probably better to concentrate on the movement in the base first and to wait for the sensation gradually to travel up to the throat, in its own time.

After a few of these breaths which are deepened and lengthened, you will find that the breath settles to a shorter inhalation, exhalation pattern. Though shorter in length, the pattern will retain a rhythm to it. The Buddha talks a lot about this process in meditation: he tells us how initially the inhalation and the exhalation are long, and yet—as there is a settling-down, whether just in sitting or in meditation—the gentle rhythm of inhalation and exhalation persists, but shortens. Through this, you can stay in that space for a while, with a quiet settled mind.

After this seated breathing, gradually let yourself come round. Gently open the eyes, but don't get up too quickly. Just be aware of your surroundings. You may want to come into *namaste* (see p. 22) and give thanks for your life and your breath, as a way of consciously ending the practice. Within the everyday life you come back into, you can be mindful of your breath—mindful of your life, mindful of how you are, where you live, how you act—without losing spontaneity.

PRACTICE 3 : KUMBHAKA—RETENTION OF THE BREATH

While retention of the breath, if done correctly, is probably the most powerful method to expand the vital force, it is not the only one. If done incorrectly, it can constrict the vital force and aggravate many diseases, just as failing to breathe causes us to faint. Through Pranayama one slows down and extends the breath so that the inner prana or higher life force can manifest. This aids in calming the mind, facilitating meditation.
Dr David Frawley, YOGA AND AYURVEDA, *Lotus Press, Twin Lakes WI, 2000*

JUST as *pranayama* is defined by some people as 'retention of the breath', so breath retention is often taught as holding the breath in, and then counting the time for which it is held. Not only is there more to *pranayama* than this, but teaching it in such a way tends to be rather forceful and contracting. It cannot be emphasized enough that if we impose a forced breathing technique onto an unnatural or disturbed breathing pattern we can constrict the flow of *prana* and disturb the mind.

There is a natural pause at the top of every inhalation and at the end of the exhalation. Before the next practice, take some time to feel these pauses in your natural rhythm. In the cycle of the breath, the inhalation is the taking-in of life, energy, love, grace. The exhalation represents surrender to life's process, and its opportunities for understanding. Whether we deem those negative or positive depends on our viewpoint. So the top of the inhalation, that transition between opening and surrender, requires a moment's pause to consider that significant process that accompanies breathing.

The pause at the end of the exhalation is a moment of choice that we have to continue life on earth.

In fact it is at this point a yogi or master (someone who has complete mastery or choice over the processes of body, mind, and emotions) would choose to pass on or die in the physical body. A *yogi* or *yogini* (feminine) believes that he or she has a certain number of breaths, and recognizes the point which is the end of them. When he or she feels it is time to go, the teacher would choose simply not to breathe in again—having informed all his or her followers what was going to happen.

The significance of the next practice, overleaf, will become apparent from this.

The only breath-retention I feel happy to practise myself and teach others, in a retreat situation, is one I was taught by Shri B. K. S. Iyengar to bring my eyes to life. He said my eyes were dull, and this particular *pranayama* brought a sparkle to them! If the eyes are the windows of the soul or an indication of how the person is within, then this *pranayama* would relieve my dullness.

This practice is like the *ujjayi pranayama* just described and illustrated, except that during the pause at the top of the inhalation the chest goes on expanding and lifting. The exhalation comes at the natural limit of that lift and opening.

To develop this practice, feel the breath come from deep in the base, in the belly, travelling up to expand the ribcage. Move the thoracic diaphragm down, fill the top chest and finally spread the throat back. Then the head wants naturally to come forward and down,

without the throat tightening. At this point, at the top of the inhalation, pause: with the breath in, go on lifting the chest up and expanding it out. When you reach the limit of that lift and opening, gently exhale. Take two or three easy breaths, and then repeat the full breath. Repeat this maybe three or four times for the first few times of doing this exercise.

In this practice you will note that although there is a pause of the breath, the body goes on moving and expanding, opening the air sacs and taking the breath deep. Do not strain at all to do this. It always needs to feel as though it is a natural movement. If this breath practice feels too demanding, but you are used to doing *asanas*, then the yoga posture *setu bandha sarvangasana* (bridge pose) will give you the required lift of the breastbone for the breathing.

The Sanskrit name for bridge pose includes the word *bandha*,

indicating that traditionally it is considered a *bandha* as well as an *asana* (posture). The position the pose puts the throat and head in, in relation to the breastbone, is exactly the same as bringing the head down in this *pranayama*. Bridge pose is helpful for any breathing practice but especially this one. You can feel the similarity in the lifting and opening of the sternum, breastbone. For further yoga postures that develop the breathing, see page 64.

This *kumbhaka* is quite a demanding *pranayama*, but worth the effort, as it brings a sense of lightness and joy. It has the effect of lifting, increasing your energy, relieving depression and dullness. It can relieve heaviness in the head. Even so, I would advise a year's regular practice of *ujjayi pranayama* before attempting this one.

Do not do this breathing practice if you are pregnant or have high blood-pressure.

CHAPTER 7
Breathing and Emotion: Fear and Trust

WHAT happens inside when you feel fear?

Fear is one of the basic reactions of all living creatures. In the animal kingdom, the adrenals—the fear-and-flight hormone glands situated

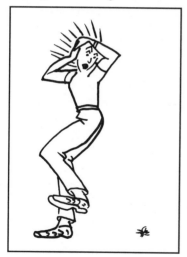

above the kidneys—go on full charge when they feel fear. The production of adrenalin enables a sudden burst of fast movement to help them to get away from the cause of the fear, or to stimulate a fight response. Humans can use this response in the adrenals too, when they need to. What is different is that humans often feel fearful in situations that they cannot run away from or from which they choose not to run away.

So what happens when we feel that surge of fear and the adrenals are ready for us either to go or to stand up and fight, and yet we don't do either of those things but nonetheless feel tremendous fear? It is often said that you can smell fear on someone. Maybe that is the adrenals pumping out adrenalin.

The adrenals sit on top of the kidneys, and the kidneys are just at the level of the lower back ribs, the left one right under the ribs, the right one a little lower down because of the location of the liver. Subjectively, it feels to me as though the kidneys tighten and grip, indeed that the adrenals tighten and grip. Is that how it feels to you: that the area of the back ribs contracts in and 'holds on', in order to keep ourselves going?

One supposedly good aspect is that this gripping and tightening of the kidneys enables us to push ourselves to the limits, maybe in ambition to prove to ourselves or someone else just how much we can do. Yet is this the root of our need to keep going excessively, to drive ourselves beyond all our natural limits? Are we afraid of stopping because of what might then come up for us, because of what we might feel?

Some of the situations we encounter are very real situations of fear. Also, we may find ourselves in situations similar to where we felt fear as a child, and thus unnecessarily bring up a host of childhood fears. For all of these, bringing our awareness to the breath, especially directing our awareness and our breath to the back of the body, relaxes us out

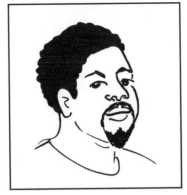

of the fear.

If, in fearful situations, we pause, breathe, and spread the back ribs, thus enabling the kidneys to relax and cease their hold, we can then come to an inner place in which we can trust that we will come through the experience. We may feel that we will be taken care of, held. Breathing itself is an action of trust that the intake of air will happen in response to the movement we make with the diaphragms. Trust is not an actual emotion, but a simple acceptance that matches completely the steadiness of the breath.

CAN you visualize, in your imagination, a situation which will make you feel fearful?

Typical examples of everyday situations that cause people fear include confrontations with particular people, for instance at work. Alternatively, classic fears might surround being in an aeroplane about to take off or land, or driving a car on a motorway in difficult traffic. These are very understandable situations that put many people in the grip of fear, but they are ones which in the main people do not run away from. Because they need to do their work or get to a certain place, or even simply because of social pressures, they feel that they have to stay with the situation.

What happens to the body, and particularly to the breath, when it feels this fear? Is there a sense of holding, of tightening of the respiratory muscles so that you don't breathe? Maybe there's even the subconscious thought that if you don't breathe, then someone might not sense you are there, so you may not get seen, you may not get hit, you may not get caught. As a schoolboy or schoolgirl, were you afraid of authority figures? Do you carry a memory that makes you tighten still when confronted, maybe recollecting times you thought you would be punished for doing something wrong?

Think about it. How does the body feel under that situation? Can you feel what the fear does to your body? What does it do to the movement of your breath through your body? Can you feel the holding that goes on in the sacrum area and the kidney area, in the throat, even across the brow?

Now, what happens if you just breathe with that, if you just open to the inhalation? See what it is like to soften with the exhalation, and thus spread into the back rib area, the kidney area? Can you gently fill those organs with *prana*, with life-force, so that they do not need to tighten? How much do you think the cells breathe in those organs that are so vital to us? By relaxing, can you let them breathe a little more?

Try to develop the sense that you can just relax out of that fear a little, that you can let go of it a little by breathing into it. Breathe into the very feeling of fear that you have in the body. Actually accept the feeling of fear, not to be overwhelmed by it, but because you can then infuse it with transforming breath. Then, really exhale and let go of the fear that you have. Develop the sense that you could really let go as you breathe out; and then let the welcome inbreath open you. Feel that you are still there, that you are still alive, your whole being is not harmed. You are still in one piece, despite those very intense feelings. Whether they are real or imagined, the breath can really release you from them; it can really move you through that fear.

Again, this process takes some staying with, some being with. It involves allowing the fear to be there in your body with you. You are not running away.

There are many supposedly irrational things that cause fear—for example, heights, spiders, confined spaces. They may seem to be trivial but there will be a real foundation to them, somewhere within: an inner pattern or memory that makes a trivial thing all-important.

We can take ourselves through the fear that comes from our subconscious by just breathing with it, in the way described. Then, we could create or feel a situation where we feel very secure: very relaxed in our surroundings, very at ease, very at peace with those around us. Better still, if we can feel that sense of security in ourselves, in who we are, or find our trust in the universe, then this is the true opposite of fear.

This process of trust again comes through pausing to take a conscious breath whenever our security is threatened. Noticing this makes us feel secure *within*.

Now think about what in our external surroundings can give us security: the safety of our own home, the protection of fences, and locks, and so on. How does that feel in our body, in our breath? Is it the same whether the securities are material, or whether they are in another person—or if, alternatively, the security seems to come from a benign universe, or the god in that universe, or in ourselves? Can we explore these considerations through our breathing?

What is the response in the body? Does it relax, does it open to your breath? Think of those areas which tend to tighten and restrict our breath when we are afraid—the solar plexus area and the throat area. When those open, when we feel comfortable in ourselves, can we breathe once again?

Now visualize a situation where you are very excited, positively so, about something that is going to happen: the return of someone you have not seen for a long time; a dream holiday; being applauded for something you have done; getting an unexpected bonus or winning a prize. What is the feeling in the body and the breath now? If it's something exciting, enticing, what happens to your whole system? It gets keyed up, yes, but is it in the same way as it is by fear? Is there a shortness of breath, a sudden inbreath, a squeal of excitement in the breath? What is the response in the diaphragm, in the breath? What is the feeling in those areas of the body that are geared up for such a response: the guts, the adrenals?

And when the exciting thing has happened—when you have enjoyed it or not as the case may be, whether it was disappointing or beyond all expectation—what's the feeling then? Is there a great sigh, a happy sigh, or is there a sigh of disappointment? What happens to the breath now, once you have relaxed from that exciting anticipation? Is it a relief? Does it feel good? Does it feel as though you can relax and breathe, or are you still holding your breath?

You may have noticed, as you created the fear situations and as you experienced the feelings and the movement in your breath, that you had a lot of memories of when you first felt this fear. You may remember how when you first felt it you tightened your body, you held your breath. If that sort of memory comes to you, and if you feel you can, let it be there: let yourself experience every aspect of that memory and notice what happens to your breath now with that memory.

You may find that the response-pattern is similar. See if you can consciously breathe yourself through that. Let the breath come in, and let it go out, through the memory. Let the breath be with that memory. Gradually, the breath will unlock the effect, the holding effect, that the memory has had on you. As usual, this may take some practice. It may take some continued repeating of the memory. Yet it will be different each time you recreate it, and there can be a sudden moment when you let go—a release, an unlocking—particularly if the happening itself was sudden, and the tightening came with it. With other experiences, maybe where the tightening was more gradual, there may need to be a much more gradual unlocking of it. That may come in phases. There is some safety built into our bodily system which prevents us unlocking these things all at once.

Do not wallow in the memories, though. Once you feel the shift in your breath, go on consciously breathing in that way, not dwelling on the memory: breathe still more deeply, more fully, more into the back body. This will bring you to the trust you need in your life's journey.

CHAPTER 8
Breathing and Emotion: Sadness and Joy

In the city of Brahman is a secret dwelling, the lotus of the heart. Within this dwelling is a space, and within that space is the fulfilment of our desires. What is within that space should be longed for and realized.

As great as the infinite space beyound is the space within the lotus of the heart. Both heaven and earth are contained in that inner space, both fire and air, sun and moon, lightning and stars. Whether we know it in this world or know it not, everything is contained in that inner space....

There is as much in that little space within the heart, as there is in the whole world outside.

Chandogya Upanishad, trans. Eknath Easwaran. London, 1987

IT IS often difficult for us to go with change. If you have strong feelings of grief and sadness or are held by the memory of someone who has died; if you are going through feelings about someone that you've lost, or feel something's ended, broken—maybe a marriage that has ended or a child that has left home—you may need to acknowledge first that such events in our lives are tremendously powerful. The rest of the time, we tend to think things will stay as they are always; but then everything changes. It is rarely easy for us to go along with this.

Many teachers will tell us that we need to feel sadness; that we need to allow the natural feeling; and yet how can we truly accept emotions which are so difficult to bear? I suggest that it helps to be aware how sadness and grief manifest in our bodies. Feel, for instance, how your shoulders tend to curve in, how your head drops, your upper back strains and your whole posture closes in on itself as it tries to contain all that sadness and grief. Let that be, for indeed we need to feel that, and first of all tell yourself that it's all right to feel grief, it's understandable that you feel sadness.

Yet at the same time, feel it with the awareness, 'How is my breath in this situation?'. Rather than trying to alter the breathing at all, go with how you are breathing. Notice it: just noticing it and going with it will change it. In the same way that life changes, your breath will change as you stay with it. Just as in nuclear physics simply to observe the situation alters it, so it is with our breath.

If we stay with that feeling of grief and sadness and indeed bring more awareness to it, almost accept it and encourage it, there is a tendency for us to feel guilty. Grief is essentially selfish and personal, and so we tend to feel guilty about that, but we can only move on into an unselfish state by first acknowledging, 'OK, this is how I feel, this is how I need to feel'. So, for the moment, really go into the experience; encompass it in all of its aspects—feeling, posture, breath, awareness. It may take time to work through the actual experience, particularly if there has been

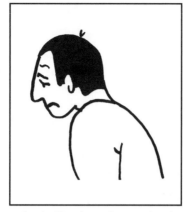

a shock. Shock tends to make the diaphragm go into spasm, and so it compounds grief. It adds another

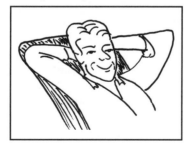

layer to what has simply to be experienced and felt. But the way forward is the same. Just absorbing the reverberations of the shock through your body by breathing into it will take you into the reality of it and yet bring you through it.

Sobbing, if that is what you need to do, is actually a very strong form of breathing, a very strong healing for the body. If gentle tears come, let them come; there could be frustration and anger at the injustice of what has happened. You may need a lot of space and solitude, and yet the process can equally be done in a group where the expression of grief is recognized. It can be worked through with a loved one, in a class situation, in a meditation; but in each case, the healing is connected with awareness of the breath and dealing with the emotion through the breath.

PRACTICE 1: MEDITATION WITH *BHAIRAVA HASTA MUDRA* (HAND MUDRAS)

THERE are actually four *mudra* practices here. The first is a version of *bhairava mudra* that lifts the heart. Sit with the spine lengthened upright, gently breathing from deep in the base, up into the belly, then into the chest and heart area. Loosely interlace the fingers (without them gripping the back of the other hand) at the level of the solar plexus or lower ribs, a few inches away from your body (see drawing below). Keep your awareness with your breathing.

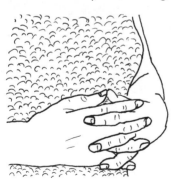

Go into your awareness. Does this *hasta mudra* lift your heart up, does it let the belly open to the breath more? Can the rib cage spread more, the whole upper body feel lighter, more lifted out of the lower body?

Meditating with this *mudra* can gradually integrate grief and sadness into our being, allowing them to be, yet taking us to the joy, seeing the blessings in all aspects of our lives.

The second mudra, the traditional *bhairava mudra,* is where the fingers of the right hand rest on the fingers of the left hand in the lap, creating a link between the two sides of the body, bringing balance and harmony. This is the more masculine *mudra,* with the right on top, and said to be more appropriate for a man. The *bhairavi mudra*, spelt with an 'i' at the end, is the feminine mudra, more appropriate for a woman, and here the fingers are the other way round: those of the left hand rest on top of those of the right hand.

The third *mudra* is *hridaya mudra* and is intended to help the heart with shock, trauma and emotional upsets and crisis. Sitting and breathing as in the first *mudra,* bring your hands onto each thigh just above the knee, palms turned upwards. Take the index finger right to the root of the thumb, bringing the middle two fingers to touch the thumb at the tips. Keep the little finger stretched out (see draw-

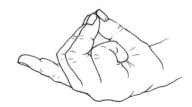

ing). Sit using this *mudra*, breathing gently, for ten to thirty minutes, feeling the calming effect it has on the mind, body and emotions.

In this *hridaya mudra* we are then reining in our ego self, connecting it to the root of our consciousness, at the same time connecting the parts of our mind that function for us in the physical day-to-day world to a greater consciousness that is whole and heart centred.

Then lie down, using what is known in yoga as *savasana* (corpse pose): flat on your back and arms relaxed a little to the sides, as shown in the drawing on p. 19. Feel the breath expanding into the body like a wave of energy touching the heart. As the breath leaves the body, you should feel a release across the chest and shoulder-girdle so that the arms relax out from the shoulders, the jaw softens, and the heart begins to lift and open. It is almost as if the arms are embracing the shock or trauma and so

MORE ON THE MUDRAS

The thumb represents *chitta* (consciousness, see p. 36).

The index finger represents *ahamkar*, the ego sense of 'I', or self-consciousness.

The middle finger represents *buddhi*, the part of the mind that discriminates and so learns from experience.

The third finger represents *manas*. *Manas* means 'instrument of thinking', the individual part of the mind that makes decisions.

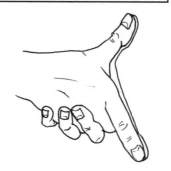

freeing the heart. With this, the holding pattern is released so that the breath can move more deeply through us.

This *mudra* and the breath-awareness that goes with it brings harmony and balance to the heart.

Lastly, the *yoni mudra*. In this, the index fingers touch at the tip and point downwards. The thumb-tips touch, pointing upwards, while the other fingers are interlaced (see drawing). This *mudra* creates a balance between mind in the head and awareness in the body, the downward fingers earthing the *ahamkar, the* upward-pointing fingers connecting *buddhi* and *manas* to *chitta* (see boxed text).

With practice of these *mudras*, you will eventually find that your fingers move into the *mudra* appropriate to your state of mind at the time. It is important that they feel relaxed, not forced or strained in any way.

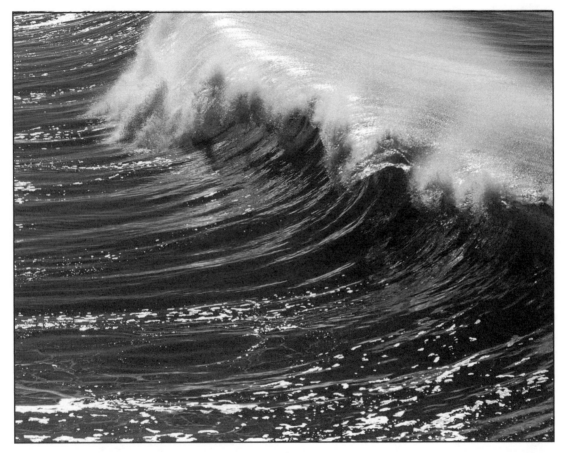

CHAPTER 9
Being Aware through the Breath

An enlightened being does not tighten, they expand their awareness every moment of time.

Ajahn Sucitto

You are awareness. Awareness is another name for you. Since you are awareness there is no need to attain or cultivate it. All that you have to do is give up being aware of other things, that is of the not-Self. If one gives up being aware of them then pure awareness remains, and that is the Self.

Sri Ramana Maharshi

IN THIS book, I have given many 'practices'. I have done this essentially to bring awareness of the breath. Although the practices have sometimes been given in relation to specific situations and emotions, the intention of the book is to help you develop awareness of the breath at all times, and the rest of the book will cover more ordinary situations. Thus we may learn to recognize how the breath is at any moment of the day, whatever we are doing, however busy we may be.

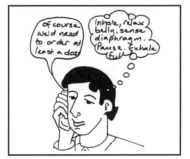

In this more focused consciousness we act, interact, live and move in awareness of who we are, how we are and what we are doing with our lives. Your breath reflects that.

WALKING

The rhythm of walking goes naturally with the rhythm of the breath. If they are allowed to, the two rhythms complement one another. If we walk with awareness of our hips moving, our feet spreading and the contact we thus make with the earth, the body opens up and the diaphragm moves, allowing the rhythm of the breath to match the rhythm of the step. As you walk, be consciously aware; because if, like most of us, you have been in the habit of holding onto your breath the rest of the time, you will probably find you still do that when walking.

So begin by being conscious of the movement of the hips, right from deep in the sacrum. Let the shoulders swing with the swing of the hips and let the breastbone lift. Soon, the breath will gradually come into a more natural rhythm; but it will need your conscious awareness of it .

There is a theory that talking as you walk disturbs the rhythm shared between the walk and the breath. The body, it is said, naturally exhales when the feet touch the ground to protect the back from impact. When we talk at the same time as walking, we interrupt this pattern. However, the risks seem more slight than the benefits of walking in company, which often may be what gets us outdoors!

Walking is often very healing and releasing for the spine, the abdominal organs and the head. Be aware of the exhalation when walking, whether alone or with a companion, because people often find it is easier to talk to one another walking. So long as we can be conscious still of our breathing, it will probably keep its rhythm. It is all the easier if the talk is heartfelt. Even if the conversation is not that easy, there is still a likelihood that through breath-awareness we can keep our balance and steadiness in whatever we need to say or want to say.

Walking balances us, tones us up and quite naturally brings awareness of the rhythm of the body and the breath. It is good to have a walk lasting at least twenty minutes once a day or more, to get this rhythm going and move the circulation. Walking stimulates the lymph glands, and all this movement in the system encourages the breath to move through our body, enabling the *prana* to bring life to it. If we are breathing fresh air, *prana*-filled air—especially easy to do by the sea, in the country, or surrounded by trees—that is going to help us open up the lungs and encourage the waking-up of the body much more.

TAKING EXERCISE

Many runners we see taking their exercise look tense and strained, especially if they are trying to force the body to do what it is not used to doing. Unless they are aware, the diaphragm may be collapsed so that they breath only with the top chest, putting incredible strain on the heart and respiratory system. A breathing practice of ten to fifteen minutes before running (see pages 20–21, on using the whole of the lungs), will help enormously if the awareness gained there is then taken into the running. Similarly, the rower (or user of a rowing machine) who remains aware and erect breathes better, but again the practice beforehand is what really helps.

DRIVING

A CAR seat, however well it is designed, does not at all encourage movement of the three diaphragms, so we need to lengthen up the spine deliberately and broaden the back. This will allow the diaphragms to open, and then we can be aware of breathing—even in tense situations such as traffic jams, hurrying to get somewhere on time, and where we have to cope with impatient or angry fellow-motorists.

A conscious inhalation and exhalation will make all the difference as to how we are dealing with such situations. We may still arrive late, but breathing through the experience will decrease much of the tension that is otherwise created. Sound, too, can be releasing of the tension that builds up, which is one unconscious reason why so many people sing along with the car stereo, enjoying the car's acoustic. The great thing is that when you are on your own in the car no-one will think anything of you opening your mouth wide! For further tips, see the Chapter 4, on sound.

FLYING

Fears around flying are very common, especially in recent times. However, the great thing to remember once we are on the plane is that we can do nothing about it except breathe! Following the instructions on page 45 for *ujjayi pranayama* will be particularly helpful, particularly at take-off and landing. It will also reduce jet-lag and the possibilities of DVT (deep vein thrombosis), which of course are also offset by simple yoga exercises you can do in cramped conditions. A *mudra* would also ground you. You might think this impossible a few thousand feet up, yet the ground is still there underneath you! The *hridaya* (heart) *mudra* would help reduce panic and fear; and simply to place the hands together in the lap, and remain conscious of them, calms the mind and settles the body.

EVERYDAY SITUATIONS SUCH AS WRITING CHEQUES

I don't suppose I am alone in finding that another stressful situation is to write a cheque when I know there is not much money in my bank account! When I am feeling a bit hard-up, I can feel that my breath tightens. I hold it in not just with my muscles but with the very feeling of there not being enough. The thought is that I can't breathe because there is not enough air, life, support, energy, money there.

At this point I now try to pause, consciously dispose of the fear and panic on an outbreath, and allow the inhalation to open my body as I write the cheque. Doing this on an inhalation encourages a sense of trust and levelness. I don't know if that should make a difference to the amount that is in my bank account, but it is good for reducing the panic! Maybe it even brings about eventually a more sensible, clear attitude to money and the energy that is behind the exchange of money. Breathing in and out are an equal exchange, so the sense of this may shift our insecurity, our fear that there is not enough.

MEETINGS

Not only business meetings but encounters with difficult neighbours, stroppy teenagers and demanding children are all situations that stress us out! If we pause in the midst of them to take an aware breath into the back of the body (see page 19) it can diffuse frustration and anger, and can avoid a reaction that later we feel to have been inappropriate.

DEALING WITH A FULL TIMETABLE

Sri Ramana Maharshi was known to say that the fuller his timetable was, the earlier he needed to rise that day to do his practice. This gave him the energy and awareness to achieve all he needed to do without stress. I can certainly echo this, although I regret I am not yet at the stage of feeling no stress at all!

Our early morning practice will make an enormous difference to how our day goes. It will affect how much energy, awareness and concentration we have, and even how much we can fit into a day, because we shall be more efficient. Enlivening breathing practices such as *nadi sodhana*, *ujjayi pranayama* and, most especially, the lifting of the breastbone given on pp. 45–6, will assist in running with a very full day.

Give yourself time within that busy day to pause and take a conscious inspiration and expiration, filling the back of the body, particularly when changing from one job to another. This will resurrect the effects of your early morning practice. At any point of the day, ask yourself, 'Am I breathing?'. You may well be surprised to notice how often you hold your breath!

A FINAL NOTE

To summarise this book, here is something to write in big letters where you'll regularly see it:

JUST
BREATHE!

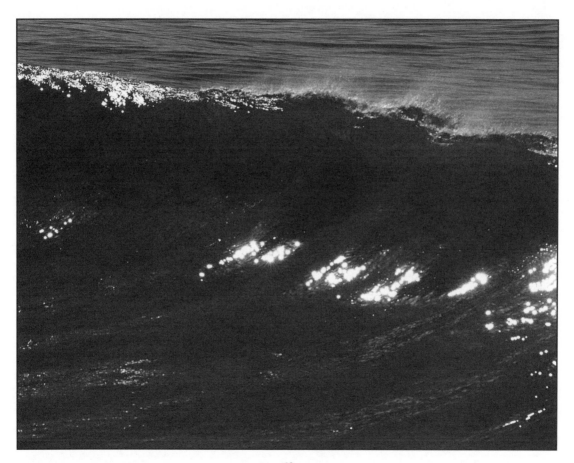

AWARENESS OF THE BREATH AND YOGA POSTURES

I WAS taught by Shri B. K. S. Iyengar that we need to practise *asana* (postures) before attempting *pranayama*. I have tried in this book to make simple breathing exercises available to people unfamiliar with yoga, but it is certainly true that if the spine is curved, the diaphragms close in and cannot move, and so we could not possibly take a full complete breath. If, through *asana*, our posture becomes more upright, and the hips and chest more open, then our breathing will naturally become fuller and more life-enhancing.

See Donna Farhi, THE BREATHING BOOK (DETAILS), for an excellent full anatomical explanation of breathing. All the postures encourage full breathing if we do not push or strain and so hold the breath to get into them. In particular, all postures that move the hips encourage the pelvic diaphragm to move. If this diaphragm moves at the base, then the other two will follow. However, below is a list of *asanas*, some of them already mentioned, that particularly help breathing:

Setu bandha sarvangasana—bridge pose—as long as the buttocks or coccyx don't tighten.

Virasana, supta virasana—hero—for opening the thoracic diaphragm. This is usually best done supported.

Tadasana—mountain—gives awareness of the diaphragms, especially the pelvic floor when the feet are alive and interacting with the earth.

Parsvottanasana—with the extension to the side known as pyramid.

Baddha konasana—caught angle (a literal translation, but known as cobbler pose)—against a wall with a blanket in lower back, opens the thoracic diaphragm.

Malasana—garland. Squatting against a wall is helpful for the breath in the back of body.

Siddhasana—pose of the powers, know as easy pose.

Padmasana—lotus pose.

All cross-legged sitting postures.

Jathara paravatanasana—lying twists with bent-leg modifications and, after practice, with straight legs, encourage opening of ribcage.

All these poses can be found in my other books, YOGA OF THE HEART (White Eagle Publishing Trust, Liss, Hampshire, 1990) and YOUR YOGA BODYMAP FOR VITALITY (Polair Publishing, London, 2003). They can also be found in LIGHT ON YOGA by B. K. S. Iyengar (HarperCollins, 2001). See also his LIGHT ON PRANAYAMA (Crossroad, 1995).

John-David Biggs's CD, THE PERFECT PRAYER, is available from Heart Yoga, 71 Rival Moor Rd., Petersfield, Hampshire GU31 4HX. A CD is also planned to use alongside this volume.